66 Firstly may I say what a user-friendly book this is. The idea of stretching i[...] has been my philosophy for a considerable length of time. As an osteopath I [...] class to patients for the last twenty years, most of whom have learned how t[...] musculoskeletal system and no longer need or seek treatment. I can thoroug[...] book with its common-sense approach to exercise. 99

Sheila Lee   Registered osteopath – clinical ergonomist, London, UK

66 Your book is outstanding. I think you came up with something, which is quite unique. 99

Dr. Harry Wallace   Professor at Palmer College of Chiropractic, USA

66 Treating your back is like dental care. Once a week brushing for an hour is not good enough, you have to do it every day for a couple of minutes. This is why I strongly recommend this book with daily exercise for a more healthy back. 99

Mark Van Straten   Nike's European Physiotherapist

66 The exercises are very easy to follow and an excellent idea. The exercises are standard back exercises that we give to people with back problems. I like the way this book encourages people to take responsibility for the care of their back. The general principles in this book seem to fit with many of the current theories about how to treat mechanical back pain. 99

Dr. Deborah Skeil   Spinal rehabilitation consultant, Department of physical medicine and rehabilitation, Christian Medical College and Hospital, Vellore, India

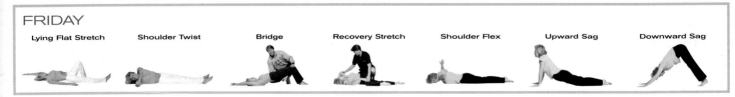

FRIDAY

| Lying Flat Stretch | Shoulder Twist | Bridge | Recovery Stretch | Shoulder Flex | Upward Sag | Downward Sag |

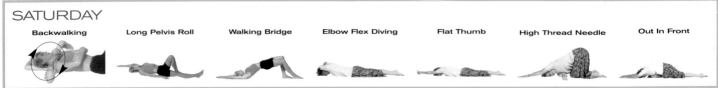

SATURDAY

| Backwalking | Long Pelvis Roll | Walking Bridge | Elbow Flex Diving | Flat Thumb | High Thread Needle | Out In Front |

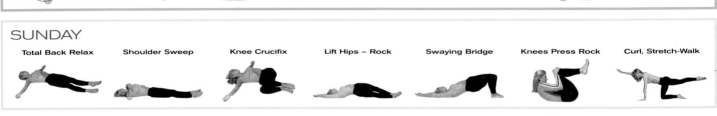

SUNDAY

| Total Back Relax | Shoulder Sweep | Knee Crucifix | Lift Hips – Rock | Swaying Bridge | Knees Press Rock | Curl, Stretch-Walk |

66 A healthy back is vital for our comfort and mobility throughout life but since we are all likely to experience some form of back pain at some time we must take precautions.

My philosophy applies whether you're a mum, an athlete, a celebrity or just a bad-back sufferer. My best advice is … stretch yourself! 99

NEIL SUMMERS   THE BACK COACH

"Since I've been using your back exercises/routine I can keep my schedule without the twinges in my back as I move through my busy day as a doctor. Being pain free through the day is a wonderful gift. Even doctors need to look after themselves. I can think of no better way than using your routine. Thank you, Neil.**"**

Dr. Sheila Phillips Santa Monica, California, USA

"The book is very impressive. As an exercise physiologist working with elite sportsmen and women I will be only too happy to recommend this excellently compiled book to them. A few minutes a day spent on exercising your back in the correct way is time well spent both for the present and future well-being.**"**

Dr. Paul Balsom Exercise physiologist, Swedish National Football Team, Stockholm, Sweden

"Excellent, clear photographs throughout the book. The structure for each exercise is very clear and very precise. By sub-dividing each exercise into starting position, movement and effect this allows the mechanics of the movement to be explained. However, even more significantly for a text of this type, it provides the reader with a rationale as to why the movement is being performed. This is very rare for a text of this type. With an ever-increasing older population, I was delighted to see that this population was catered for in this book. Overall, I would highly recommend this text for individuals of all ages and fitness levels.**"**

Vish Unnithan Ph.D. Professor of Exercise & Sport Science, University of San Francisco, USA

Your Daily Routine

MONDAY

Spine Lengthener	Knee Press	Curled Ball On Side	Forearm Press-up	Extended Thumb	Sky Diving	Shoulder Stretch

TUESDAY

Straight Stretch Hold	Double Knee Press	Face Up Chest Lift	Rock And Wrap	Chest Raise	Forearm Walk	Curled Ball

WEDNESDAY

Back Loosener	Lumbar Press	Neck Press	Pelvis Roll	Side Bends	Ab Strengtheners	Half Twist
		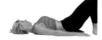				

THURSDAY

All-fours	Shoulder Tilt	Thread Needle	Double Arm Raise	Hips Lift	Low Ab Toner	Curl and Stretch

Introducing our team

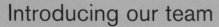

Sharron Davies is a former Olympic swimmer, Gold Medal athlete and now TV presenter. Sharron started international swimming at the age of ten and competed for her country in three Olympics in three different decades, a career spanning some twenty years. After winning medals in every major championship she retired in the mid Nineties to pursue a new career in broadcasting. She has a young family and manages to combine motherhood with a full time profession, as well as maintaining a high level of personal fitness. After a two-year appearance on Gladiators, a very physical TV show, she sustained a knee injury, which led to back problems that she now keeps under control with the use of these simple and effective back exercises.

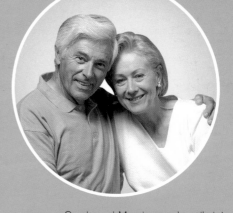

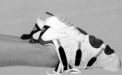

Carole and Maurice are happily into the Third Age and they are doing just fine. They really enjoyed working through this new Seven-Day Exercise program. And, as you will see, they came through looking every bit as supple as Sharron.

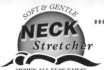

NECK *Stretcher*

"WHEN ALL ELSE FAILS"

...The drug-free way to lose that headache!

The Soft & Gentle Neckstretcher is designed to cradle the neck along the base of the skull, keeping the head and spinal column in the correct alignment.

Shaped in the reverse image of the curvature of the neck. Thumb-like nodules apply pressure to the muscles and acupressure points on either side of the spine. The weight of the head gives gentle traction to the neck, while the nodules have a massaging effect, designed to relieve muscular aches and tension.

Soft & Gentle Neckstretcher will soothe away pain & stress...

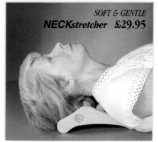

SOFT & GENTLE **NECKstretcher £29.95**

Neil Summers says, "the Neckstretcher fights all neck tension-related conditions, including computer fatigue". Most people in sedentary occupations will experience tension in the upper shoulders. This is often exacerbated by bad posture, particularly for those at desk-bound jobs or those who spend many hours driving.

"Within minutes my neck pain had disappeared. I used to suffer with headaches and bad neck pain but now find the Neckstretcher invaluable in relieving my headaches."

Doris. 62. Retired. Yorkshire

The Backstretcher and the Neckstretcher can be ideally used together for multiple benefits in one session.

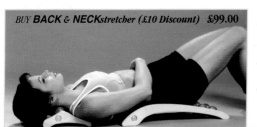

BUY **BACK** *&* **NECK**stretcher *(£10 Discount)* **£99.00**

COMFORTABLE

NECK FULLY SUPPORTED

STABLE & SAFE

BUILT TO LAST A LIFETIME

80-90% of all backache is low back pain.

Until now Backstretching devices have not made contact with this part of the body. During sitting particularly the lower back is stressed and strained in a way which 'squashes' all the discs. Using the Backstretcher in this way is the perfect antidote. It counters the sitting position exactly and eases the strain on the muscles & ligaments, reversing the pressure felt in this area after years of compression. Sitting is without doubt the 'big bad nasty'.

The 'soft & gentle' Backstretcher is without doubt the solution.

Buying the Backstretcher and the Neckstretcher together qualifies you to a £10 discount

ORDERING HAS NEVER BEEN EASIER...
0870 753 3765

SPORTS *Stretcher*

"WHEN ALL ELSE FAILS"

At last a "Sports" Stretcher for the fit & healthy

The difference between the 'Soft & Gentle' Backstretcher and the larger 'Sports' version is that the 'Soft & Gentle' Backstretcher was designed to help individuals with back problems.

If a person is in pain or has anything wrong with their back then the product to choose is the award winning 'Soft & Gentle' Backstretcher. Healthy individuals with no history of backache can use the Sports version to increase suppleness. Athletes use it to increase their flexibility. Gymnastic individuals or people familiar with exercising and who are still 'working out' use it as the ultimate in "warm up" or "cool down" stretching. If you are a stiff or inflexible individual by nature then the 'Soft & Gentle' Backstretcher is the version for you. **If your gym does not have a Sportstretcher, here's your chance to get your own!**

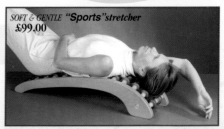

SOFT & GENTLE **"Sports"stretcher £99.00**

About the author

Neil Summers was an international lecturer in
Physical Education. He formerly served with
the British Royal Marine Special Forces,
and has a Masters Degree from
Springfield College, Mass, USA

He now works as a health educator,
advising major international corporations
exactly how to design products for a healthy life.
One of Neil's more famous inventions is the
Backstretcher, which was selected as British Invention of
the Year, making Neil the British Inventor of the Year 1995.

As a Body Coach he has helped national heads of state,
politicians, sports stars, and a host of American, Japanese,
and European celebrities.

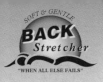
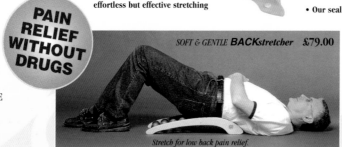
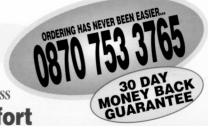

To Fiona and our three beautiful girls Francesca, Georgina and Charlotte in the hope that you are always blessed with health, love and happiness.

Published in Great Britain in 2001 by EnanefPress, Beechwood House, King George's Hill, Dorking, RH5 6JW Tel: 0870 753 3765

A CIP catalogue record for this book is available from the British Library

ISBN 0-9538123-1-6

Produced by EnanefPress, Editor: Michael Powell, Design: Andrew Clark, Photography: William Taylor.
Printed and bound in HK

Please read the instructions in this book thoroughly and follow them carefully.
If in any doubt about the appropriateness of this exercise routine, please consult with your doctor before using this book.
This routine is not intended as a substitute for professional medical care; it may not be suitable for all people.
Again, if in any doubt please consult your doctor. If you feel pain or dizziness, stop using this routine.

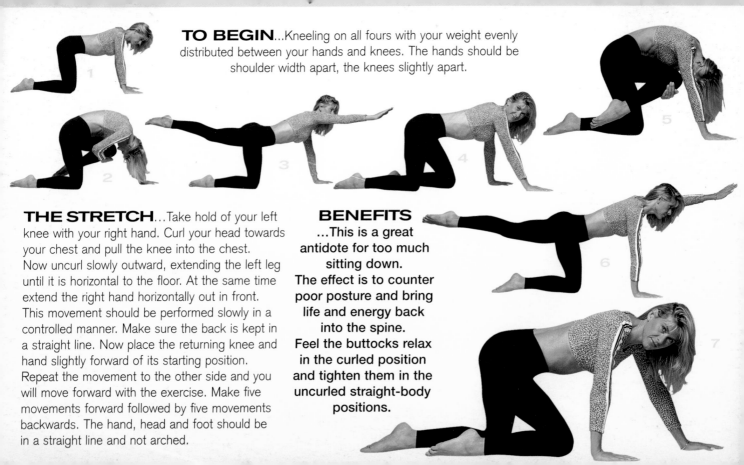

TO BEGIN...Kneeling on all fours with your weight evenly distributed between your hands and knees. The hands should be shoulder width apart, the knees slightly apart.

THE STRETCH...Take hold of your left knee with your right hand. Curl your head towards your chest and pull the knee into the chest. Now uncurl slowly outward, extending the left leg until it is horizontal to the floor. At the same time extend the right hand horizontally out in front. This movement should be performed slowly in a controlled manner. Make sure the back is kept in a straight line. Now place the returning knee and hand slightly forward of its starting position. Repeat the movement to the other side and you will move forward with the exercise. Make five movements forward followed by five movements backwards. The hand, head and foot should be in a straight line and not arched.

BENEFITS
...This is a great antidote for too much sitting down. The effect is to counter poor posture and bring life and energy back into the spine. Feel the buttocks relax in the curled position and tighten them in the uncurled straight-body positions.

CONTENTS

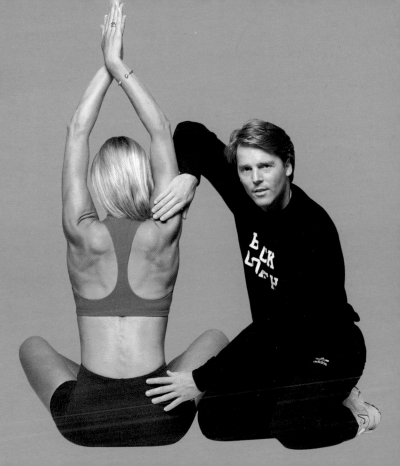

Introducing our team

About the Author

Foreword

Introduction

Backstretching

...to relieve backache

...to stay in shape

BACK IN SHAPE:

"7 Minutes" - to a healthy back and toned stomach.

Day by Day Routine

Monday

Tuesday

Wednesday

Thursday

Friday

Saturday

Sunday

The Back Coach's Equipment Guide.

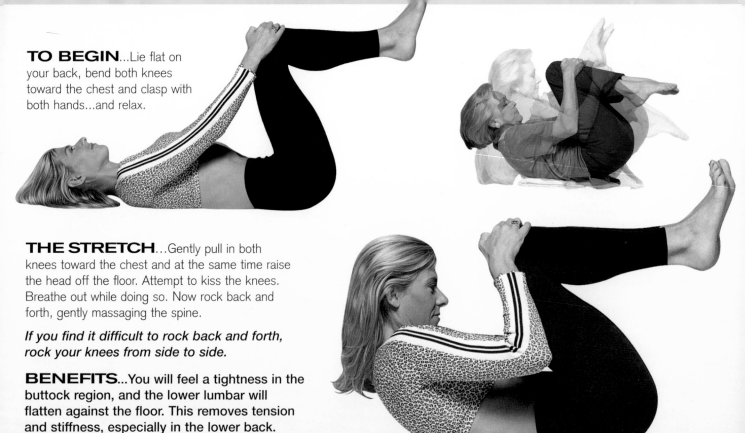

TO BEGIN...Lie flat on your back, bend both knees toward the chest and clasp with both hands...and relax.

THE STRETCH...Gently pull in both knees toward the chest and at the same time raise the head off the floor. Attempt to kiss the knees. Breathe out while doing so. Now rock back and forth, gently massaging the spine.

If you find it difficult to rock back and forth, rock your knees from side to side.

BENEFITS...You will feel a tightness in the buttock region, and the lower lumbar will flatten against the floor. This removes tension and stiffness, especially in the lower back.

Foreword

We are proud owners of a single spine and it will have to serve us a whole lifetime. But we do not take very good care of this precious and unique device! It is estimated that more than 80% of the population will suffer from back pain. But, strikingly, in about 90% of those cases, a precise cause of the suffering will not be found despite all the investigative processes of modern medicine. Most problems are functional problems. There is nothing wrong with the back, it is just being misused. The back needs to move. The loads on the discs need to be relieved and the back muscles need to relax. Neil Summers has brought together in this book a number of simple exercises, which will help you achieve those goals. The book is easy to read and easy to use. A few minutes of care for your back every day will ensure a friendlier relationship with your spine!

I recommend this book not only to back sufferers but also as a preventative tool to all those who want to keep their back in shape.

Dr. Marek Szpalski   Consultant in Orthopaedic Surgery, Associate Professor, Free University of Brussels, Belgium.   Adjunct Assistant Professor, Vanderbilt University, Nashville, USA.   Senior scientist, Hospital for Joint Diseases, New York University, USA.
Co-editor of Lumbar Segmental Instability (Lippincott, 1998)

Low back pain remains a problem for many of us. In fact, about 75% of us will have a significant episode at some time in our life. Neil Summers has developed a series of exercises, which have some support in laboratory studies we have conducted. The book is beautifully illustrated and easy to follow. It is recommended to the chronic low back sufferer who has no serious medical condition – this represents most people with lower back pain!

Malcolm Pope DrMedSc, PhD   Professor and Chair of Health and Safety, Department of Biomedical Physics and Director of the Liberty Centre, University of Aberdeen.   Adjunct Professor, University of Patras, Greece.   Adjunct Professor, University of Iowa, USA.

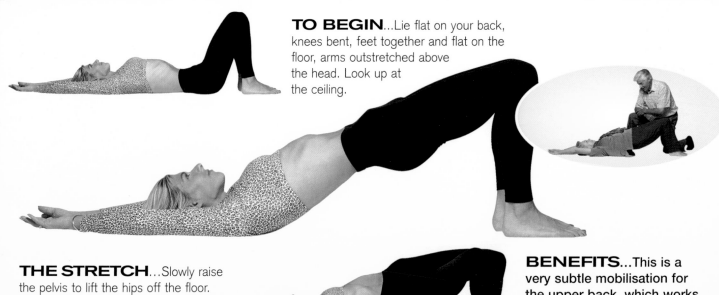

TO BEGIN...Lie flat on your back, knees bent, feet together and flat on the floor, arms outstretched above the head. Look up at the ceiling.

THE STRETCH...Slowly raise the pelvis to lift the hips off the floor. Keep your weight on heels and shoulders to form a bridge. Breathe normally. Now slowly move your pelvis a few inches over to the left, and then back to the right. Set up a gentle swaying motion. Keep the neck flat against the floor.

BENEFITS...This is a very subtle mobilisation for the upper back, which works out deep-seated muscle tension. Keeping the neck long and lengthened is an integral part of a healthy spine.

Introduction

You will not find a more superb piece of machinery than your body. Unfortunately, it is seldom allowed to function in the way for which it was designed. The result, for the majority of us, is that we are rarely free from pain.

We constantly overload the back with tasks and habits that lead to poor posture. As we age, our back bends forwards and shortens and we lose the all-round flexibility that we had in our youth. Most of our adult days are spent flexed forward, crumpled in a forward bending position, hunched over our everyday tasks.
So insidious is this forward 'pull' of the head that we do not even notice it is happening. What makes things worse is that most of us have stopped using our bodies to move in any dynamic or athletic way at all.
But if we do not let our back perform the varied array of movements it is capable of, we condemn ourselves to a life of aches and pains.

So, what can you DO about YOUR back?

My answer lies in this simple proposition – TAKE THE WEIGHT OFF YOUR SPINE. Do not allow your spine, and the spaces between the vertebrae, to become overly compressed. Learn to elongate the vertebral column with the daily exercises demonstrated in this book. I believe this is the best way to counter the miseries of backache. If you can reverse the trend of a lifetime and take the weight off your back during the daytime, you will witness the rebirth of your spine.

TO BEGIN....Lie flat on your back, extend both arms above your head, legs stretched out.

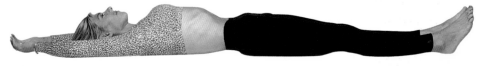

THE STRETCH...Taking the weight on the shoulders and the heels, lift your hips up off the floor to create a mini arch. Look up at the ceiling. Breathe naturally. Gently sway the hips a few inches from side to side.

BENEFITS...Feel the massage effect in the shoulders and the upper back. You should feel your buttocks tighten and a stretch in the rib cage as well as a general lengthening effect along the whole of the spine. Tension and stiffness in the shoulder region are slowly released.

Back Stretching – to relieve backache

The good news, we are told, is that exercise is once more in fashion for the treatment of backache. However, this is only partly a good thing. In fact, not all exercise is good for the back – and certain forms of exercise are actually bad for it. That is why so many people merely make their back problems worse by exercising in the wrong way, and this in turn helps to perpetuate the myth that once you have a bad back, you will always have one. It does not need to be this way. By exercising in the correct way, stretching and strengthening your back, your aches and pains will significantly diminish, resulting in a back that functions as it should…pain free.

As a remedy for back sufferers, bed-rest has been the most trusted friend of doctors through the centuries. However, we must realise why this should be so. In terms of body positioning, it is the act of going horizontal which helps us. By taking up this position, as we do each time we go to bed, we immediately remove the stresses and strains on the spine caused by the compressional effects of gravity. Literally, we take the weight off the spaces between the vertebrae. This is heaven to the damaged joint. It arrests further damage and allows the joint time to recover, repair and recuperate.

The whole story of the human back is very simple really. The back wants to move as it was designed to move. It yearns to be free to move again – fully elongated lengthways. You only have to look at our friends in the animal kingdom. Animals naturally open out their bodies when they move, and in the process reap the benefits of fully extended stretching, as opposed to the compressive forward-bending kind of movements that we are constantly making.

The weekly routine, which follows, is designed specifically to counter poor posture, muscle spasm and restricted movements, and to allow the spine once again to function properly. For more than 10 years I myself suffered from a severe back condition. I studied ways to correct my own spinal curvature and carefully developed a repeating Seven-Day Exercise Routine. Now I have good posture and have been pain-free since using this routine. In solving my own problems, I also discovered a way to give real hope to other back-pain sufferers.

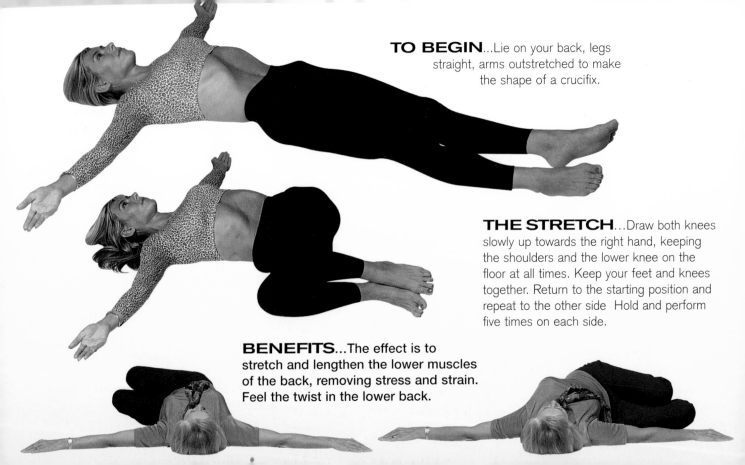

TO BEGIN...Lie on your back, legs straight, arms outstretched to make the shape of a crucifix.

THE STRETCH...Draw both knees slowly up towards the right hand, keeping the shoulders and the lower knee on the floor at all times. Keep your feet and knees together. Return to the starting position and repeat to the other side Hold and perform five times on each side.

BENEFITS...The effect is to stretch and lengthen the lower muscles of the back, removing stress and strain. Feel the twist in the lower back.

Back Stretching – to stay in shape

Damage to the joints can occur in all kinds of ways – through sporting injuries, car accidents, and hereditary complaints, through wear and tear or even the slightest of sudden, awkward movements. Once damaged, the joints in the spine suffer a constant and never-ending downward pressure, which serves only to make the situation worse. Every day during each one of the 14-16 hours a day we spend simply sitting or standing, we allow the forces of gravity to push down on us. The average adult head weighs between 11 and 13 pounds, and for all those 14 hours or more each day, it is squashing down on everything beneath it.

THE SAFEST AND MOST EFFECTIVE BACK EXERCISES ARE THOSE CARRIED OUT WHEN THE BODY IS IN A HORIZONTAL PLANE.

Lying down is the most comfortable position for a person with backache. The vertebrae are 'suspended', with no postural stress, and so they can relax and the sufferer's pain is relieved. Lying down produces the least pressure on the spaces between the vertebrae, which is why the back actually lengthens during sleep.
Relieved of weight-bearing pressures, the discs are allowed to re-hydrate, repair and recover.

My golden rule is this: LIE DOWN TO DO BACK EXERCISES.

Doing exercises in the horizontal plane allows the spine to be stretched without the weight of the body exerting compression on any joints, which are damaged, or not functioning properly. The exercises in this book are safe, simple and ultra-friendly. It doesn't matter if you are an injured athlete in your twenties or a grandmother in your seventies, you too can safely and successfully do these exercises.

Horizontal stretching gently opens out and straightens that bent or hunched-over back, giving you a mobile and fully functioning spine. **It is all unbelievably simple – so simple - it really works.**

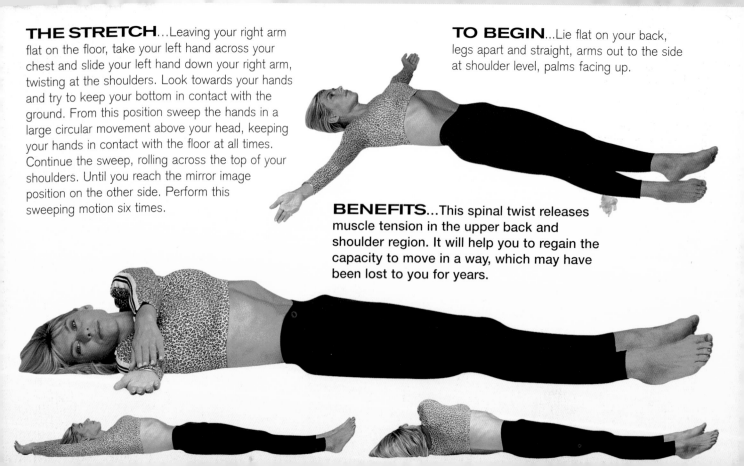

THE STRETCH...Leaving your right arm flat on the floor, take your left hand across your chest and slide your left hand down your right arm, twisting at the shoulders. Look towards your hands and try to keep your bottom in contact with the ground. From this position sweep the hands in a large circular movement above your head, keeping your hands in contact with the floor at all times. Continue the sweep, rolling across the top of your shoulders. Until you reach the mirror image position on the other side. Perform this sweeping motion six times.

TO BEGIN...Lie flat on your back, legs apart and straight, arms out to the side at shoulder level, palms facing up.

BENEFITS...This spinal twist releases muscle tension in the upper back and shoulder region. It will help you to regain the capacity to move in a way, which may have been lost to you for years.

BACK IN SHAPE

"7 Minutes" - to a healthy back and toned stomach.

NEIL SUMMERS

WITH

SHARRON DAVIES MBE.
Enanef Press

THE BACK COACH'S DAILY ROUTINE.

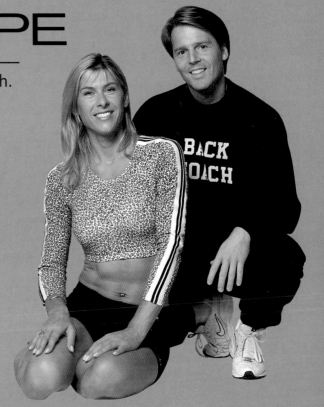

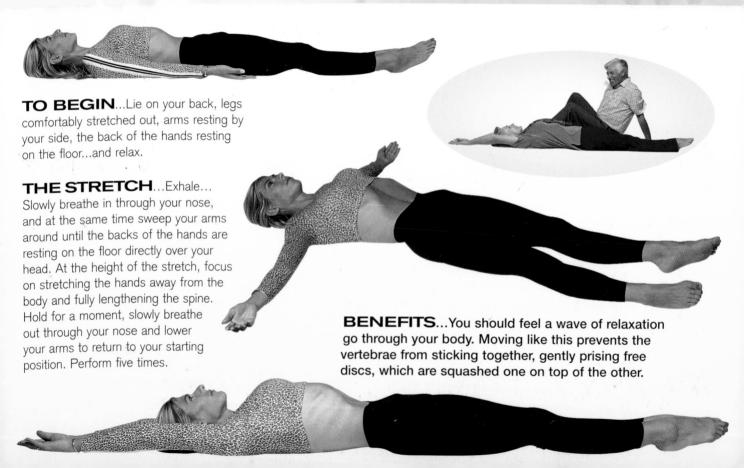

TO BEGIN...Lie on your back, legs comfortably stretched out, arms resting by your side, the back of the hands resting on the floor...and relax.

THE STRETCH...Exhale... Slowly breathe in through your nose, and at the same time sweep your arms around until the backs of the hands are resting on the floor directly over your head. At the height of the stretch, focus on stretching the hands away from the body and fully lengthening the spine. Hold for a moment, slowly breathe out through your nose and lower your arms to return to your starting position. Perform five times.

BENEFITS...You should feel a wave of relaxation go through your body. Moving like this prevents the vertebrae from sticking together, gently prising free discs, which are squashed one on top of the other.

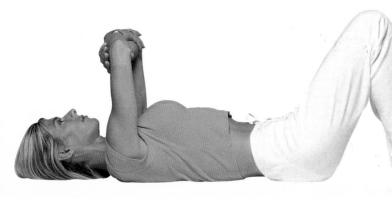

TO BEGIN…Lie on your back, knees bent, feet flat on the floor. Loosely hold your forearms in front of your chest, elbows pointing straight up. Look up at the ceiling.

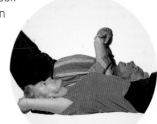

THE STRETCH…Breathe in…

Exhale and tighten your stomach muscles as you bring your arms back over your head until the forearms are resting on the floor. Relax for a moment, breathe in…. exhale tightening your tummy muscles,

then bring your arms forward over your head, through the starting position to rest on your tummy. And relax. Perform the whole sequence slowly five times. Make all movements smooth, controlled and continuous.

BENEFITS…You will feel the stretch in your rib cage and along the full length of the spine. The spine will lengthen as you relax. This simple stretch helps to open up/de-squash or decompress the spongy discs, prising them free and helping the spine to move and function as it was designed. Exhaling and tensing the tummy muscles helps to firm this area. The spine is lengthened and the stomach muscles are toned.

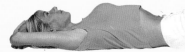

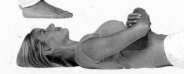

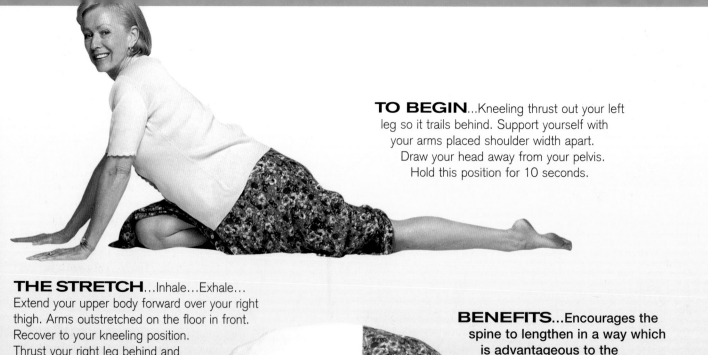

TO BEGIN...Kneeling thrust out your left leg so it trails behind. Support yourself with your arms placed shoulder width apart. Draw your head away from your pelvis. Hold this position for 10 seconds.

THE STRETCH...Inhale...Exhale... Extend your upper body forward over your right thigh. Arms outstretched on the floor in front. Recover to your kneeling position. Thrust your right leg behind and repeat the stretch on the opposite side.

BENEFITS...Encourages the spine to lengthen in a way which is advantageous to the sedentary individual.

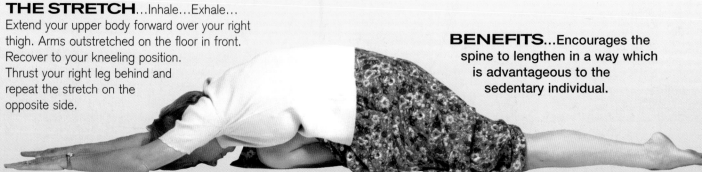

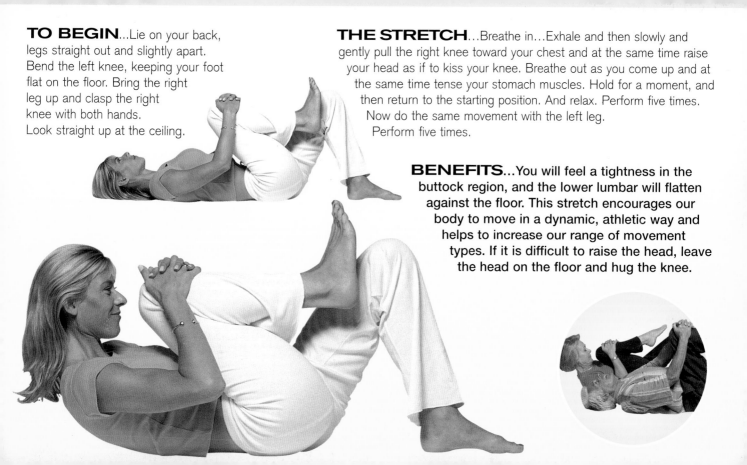

TO BEGIN...Lie on your back, legs straight out and slightly apart. Bend the left knee, keeping your foot flat on the floor. Bring the right leg up and clasp the right knee with both hands. Look straight up at the ceiling.

THE STRETCH...Breathe in...Exhale and then slowly and gently pull the right knee toward your chest and at the same time raise your head as if to kiss your knee. Breathe out as you come up and at the same time tense your stomach muscles. Hold for a moment, and then return to the starting position. And relax. Perform five times. Now do the same movement with the left leg. Perform five times.

BENEFITS...You will feel a tightness in the buttock region, and the lower lumbar will flatten against the floor. This stretch encourages our body to move in a dynamic, athletic way and helps to increase our range of movement types. If it is difficult to raise the head, leave the head on the floor and hug the knee.

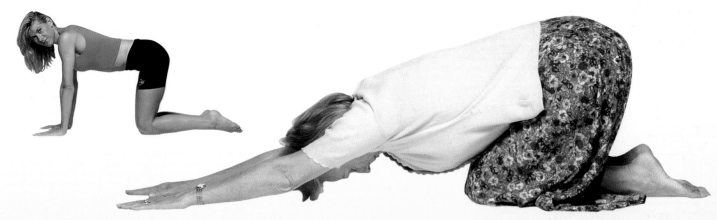

TO BEGIN...Kneeling...

sit back...reach forward, arms shoulder width apart to take up the 'cat stretch'. Keep your head low and buttocks high.

THE STRETCH...Take your right hand and

place the back of the hand underneath your left elbow. Slide out the back of the hand away from the body at 90°. Hold for 5 seconds. Recover to your original starting position and repeat sliding your left hand underneath your right elbow.

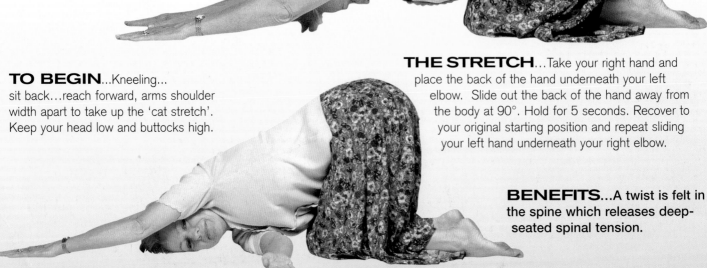

BENEFITS...A twist is felt in

the spine which releases deep-seated spinal tension.

TO BEGIN...Lie on your right hip with legs slightly bent, lower arm resting under your head, left arm resting on hip.

THE STRETCH...Breathe in, exhale and curl your head forward whilst bringing your knees up to meet the head, remembering to draw your knees up using your tummy muscles. Hold this tight curled position. Relax once in this final curled position and breathe normally. Hold for a few seconds. Uncurl, roll over onto left hip and repeat this movement on the other side.

BENEFITS...Particularly good for releasing tightness in the lower lumbar. Relieves the pressure on the discs due to the stacking effect, which occurs during excessive standing and sitting. As you relax, you should be able to curl up tighter, using your breathing to encourage further stretch. As you exhale curl further.

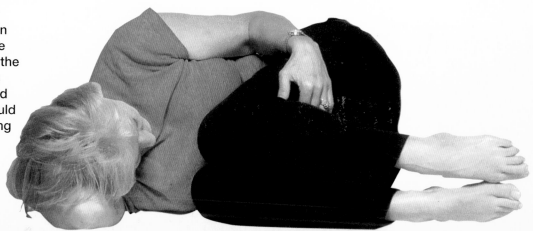

TO BEGIN...Lie face down, forehead resting lightly on the floor. Place your hands by your side. Legs straight out...and relax.

THE STRETCH...Take your left hand and extend your left thumb down to your spine.

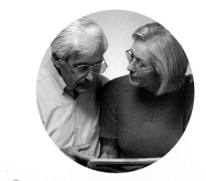

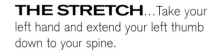

Now extend your left arm out in front. Extend your right thumb away from your body creating a long straight stretch. Do the same with the right hand and thumb. Repeat twice each hand.

BENEFITS...Feel the lengthening of the whole spine. Vertebrae that have been jammed up together all day are gently eased apart.

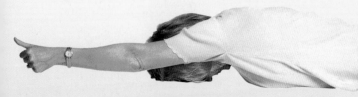

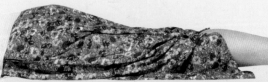

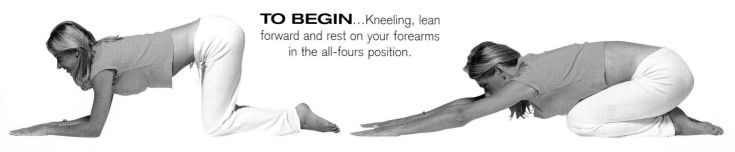

TO BEGIN…Kneeling, lean forward and rest on your forearms in the all-fours position.

THE STRETCH…Breathe in…Exhale tensing your tummy muscles and try to sit back on your heels, and at the same time straighten your arms out in front of you. Each time you exhale sink deeper into this stretch. Now bring the arms back to rest on the forearms, moving your upper body forward. As you do so, slide the forearms forward and lower the pelvis slowly to the ground. (You may need to adjust your forearms to be in line with your head as you move forward). As you stretch in this position tighten your stomach muscles. Perform the complete movement five times in a continuous flowing sequence.

BENEFITS…You should feel your head stretching away from your pelvis. Concentrate on lengthening the spine and drawing the head away from the pelvis. This movement helps the spine to become supple and strong.

TO BEGIN...Lie face down. Lightly resting your forehead on the floor. Clasp your fingers behind your neck. Place your elbows on the floor.

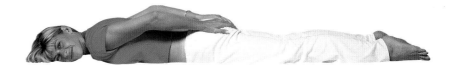

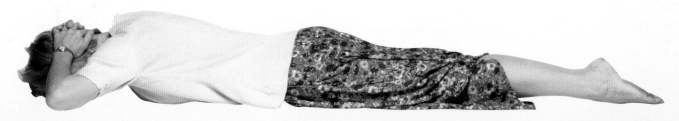

THE STRETCH...Inhale...Exhale...Raise your elbows off the floor 'scrunch' up your shoulders. Hold at the top. And relax. Return elbows to the starting position. Repeat 5 times.

BENEFITS...Great stretch for releasing tension related headaches. The tensing followed by relaxing of the back muscles has an excellent toning effect, leaving supple relaxed shoulders.

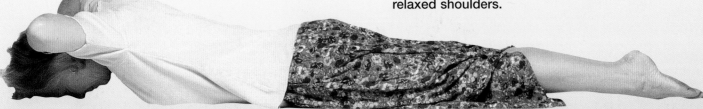

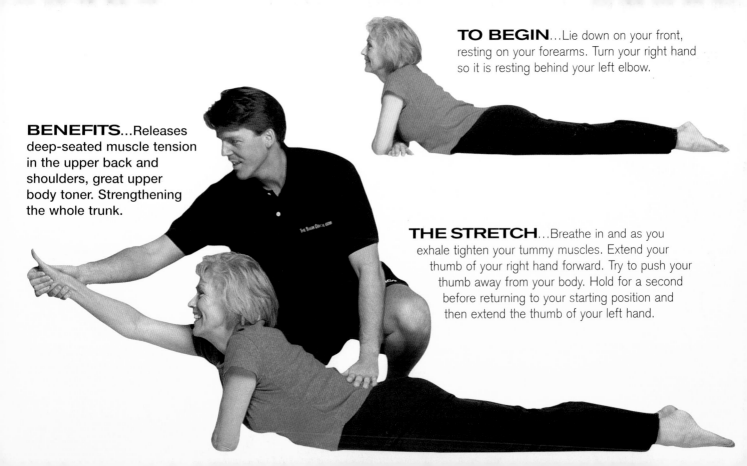

TO BEGIN…Lie down on your front, resting on your forearms. Turn your right hand so it is resting behind your left elbow.

BENEFITS…Releases deep-seated muscle tension in the upper back and shoulders, great upper body toner. Strengthening the whole trunk.

THE STRETCH…Breathe in and as you exhale tighten your tummy muscles. Extend your thumb of your right hand forward. Try to push your thumb away from your body. Hold for a second before returning to your starting position and then extend the thumb of your left hand.

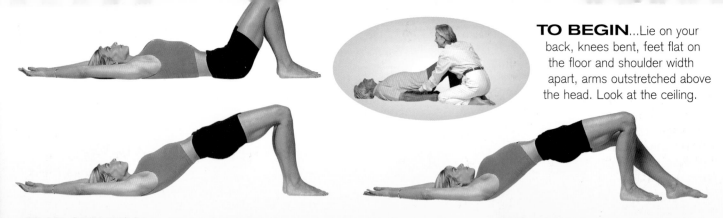

TO BEGIN…Lie on your back, knees bent, feet flat on the floor and shoulder width apart, arms outstretched above the head. Look at the ceiling.

THE STRETCH…Inhale…Exhale…Tighten your tummy muscles. Slowly raise the pelvis to lift the hips off the floor, keeping the neck flat against the floor. Keep the weight on the heels and shoulders to form a bridge. Breathe normally. Now slowly move first one leg a few inches away from your pelvis and then the other. Walk the legs out away from the body a few inches then walk them back to the starting position. The pelvis sways from side to side. Remember to retract the chin and flatten the neck against the floor.

Little movements are better than no movements.

BENEFITS…This movement massages the very top of the upper back, working out deep-seated muscle tension. Stretching the back in a lengthways direction eases the joints apart. The result is to remove weight and pressure from the damaged joints.

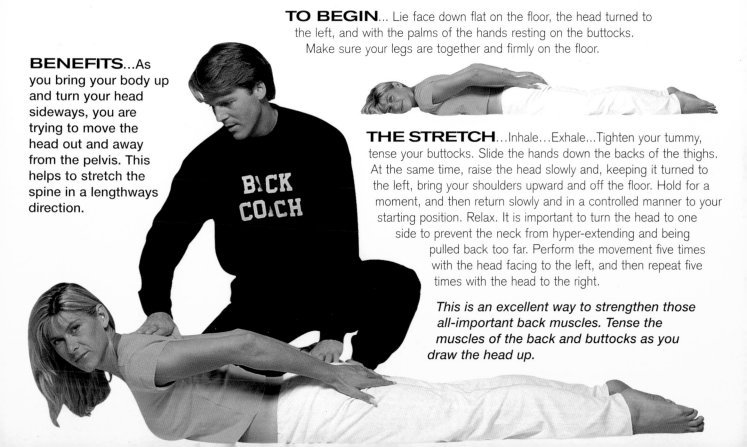

BENEFITS...As you bring your body up and turn your head sideways, you are trying to move the head out and away from the pelvis. This helps to stretch the spine in a lengthways direction.

TO BEGIN... Lie face down flat on the floor, the head turned to the left, and with the palms of the hands resting on the buttocks. Make sure your legs are together and firmly on the floor.

THE STRETCH...Inhale...Exhale...Tighten your tummy, tense your buttocks. Slide the hands down the backs of the thighs. At the same time, raise the head slowly and, keeping it turned to the left, bring your shoulders upward and off the floor. Hold for a moment, and then return slowly and in a controlled manner to your starting position. Relax. It is important to turn the head to one side to prevent the neck from hyper-extending and being pulled back too far. Perform the movement five times with the head facing to the left, and then repeat five times with the head to the right.

This is an excellent way to strengthen those all-important back muscles. Tense the muscles of the back and buttocks as you draw the head up.

BACK COACH

TO BEGIN...Lie flat on your back, the left arm outstretched over the head, the right arm relaxed by your side.

At the same time the right leg is stretched out and the left leg is bent, foot flat on the floor.

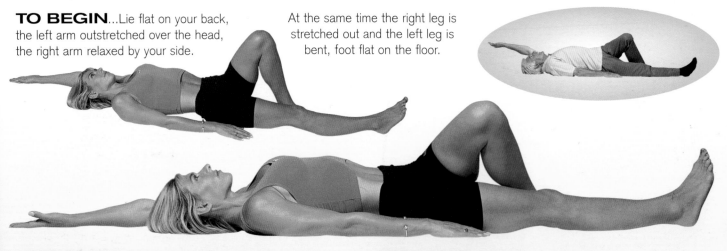

THE STRETCH...Inhale...Exhale...Tighten your tummy muscles. In this position you should aim to stretch the arm and leg further away from the body. Leading with the left knee, sway it six inches over the centre line of the body, and let it sway back to its starting position. Sway across for six movements. Change leg and repeat the movement on the other side.

BENEFITS...Feel a rocking motion around your pelvis. Rocking in this way gently loosens up the lower lumbar. Stretching in this way prevents the spine from sticking together, gently prising free discs which are squashed one on top of the other.

The minute you stop moving, the body starts to seize up. Keep the mobility and range of movement you have by stretching every day.

TO BEGIN…Lie face down, lightly resting your forehead on the floor. Lace your fingertips together behind your back – resting on your buttocks.

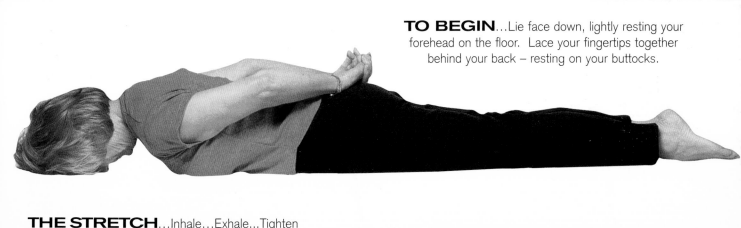

THE STRETCH…Inhale…Exhale…Tighten your tummy muscles. Keeping your arms straight. Raise your hands outwards and upwards. Hold at the top of the stretch. Return your hands to the starting position under control. And relax.
Repeat five times.

BENEFITS…This is a strong upper back muscle tension releaser. The strength and flexibility quickly develops in the shoulder muscles and the tension dissipates. Returns the shoulders to their pre-tension days, and regains lost flexibility.

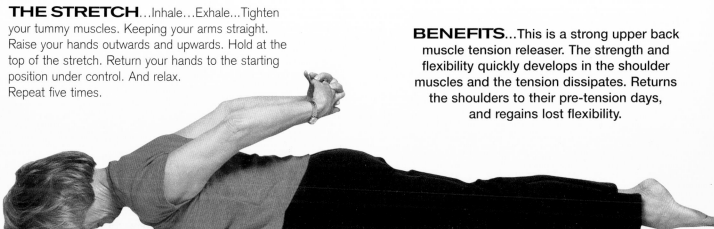

TO BEGIN...Lie flat on your back, knees bent, and feet flat on the floor. Lightly hold your forearms, resting on the floor above your head.

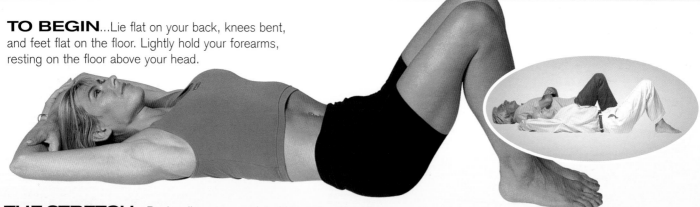

THE STRETCH...Backwalking is completed by circling the arms in a sweeping motion. Inhale...Exhale...Tighten your tummy muscles. Move the arms first to the left, sweeping down over the tummy and on up the right hand side. Sweep the arms round in a circular fashion, making large circles with the interlocked forearms. Circle five times. Repeat the process with the forearms moving in the opposite direction. Again circle 5 times.

BENEFITS...Lengthways stretching helps to free each vertebra from impacting with the one below. This stretch helps to spread out the impacted vertebrae, easing pressure in the damaged area.

If you only do one exercise before you go to bed each night, it should be this one.

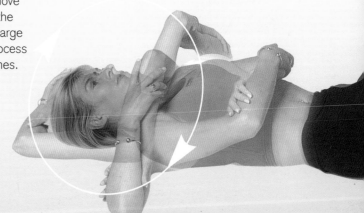

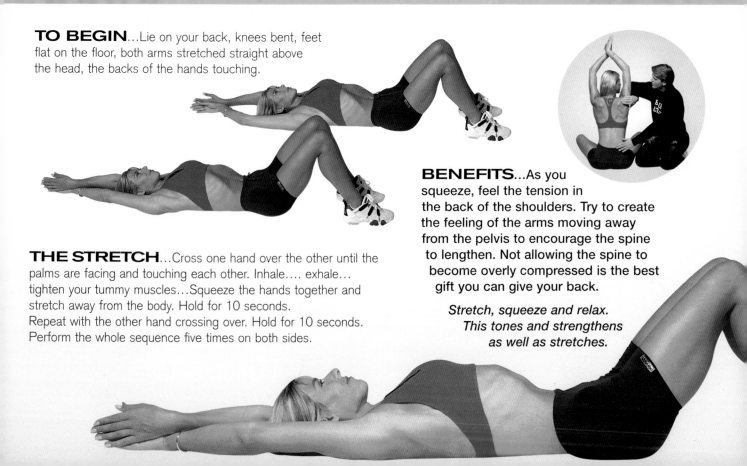

TO BEGIN…Lie on your back, knees bent, feet flat on the floor, both arms stretched straight above the head, the backs of the hands touching.

THE STRETCH…Cross one hand over the other until the palms are facing and touching each other. Inhale…. exhale… tighten your tummy muscles…Squeeze the hands together and stretch away from the body. Hold for 10 seconds.
Repeat with the other hand crossing over. Hold for 10 seconds.
Perform the whole sequence five times on both sides.

BENEFITS…As you squeeze, feel the tension in the back of the shoulders. Try to create the feeling of the arms moving away from the pelvis to encourage the spine to lengthen. Not allowing the spine to become overly compressed is the best gift you can give your back.

Stretch, squeeze and relax.
This tones and strengthens
as well as stretches.

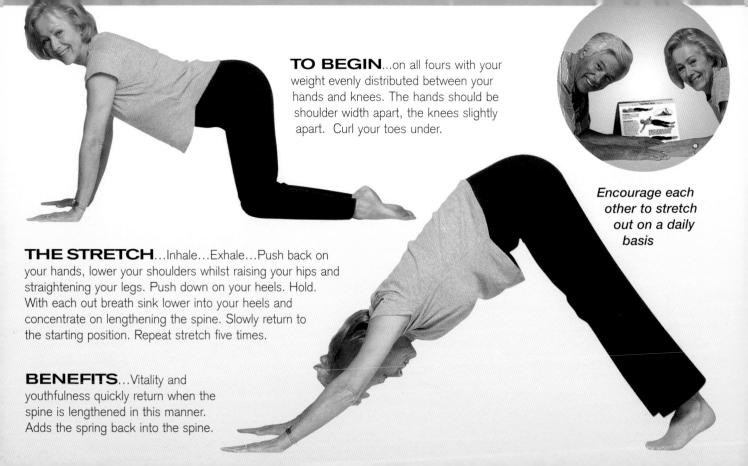

TO BEGIN...on all fours with your weight evenly distributed between your hands and knees. The hands should be shoulder width apart, the knees slightly apart. Curl your toes under.

Encourage each other to stretch out on a daily basis

THE STRETCH...Inhale...Exhale...Push back on your hands, lower your shoulders whilst raising your hips and straightening your legs. Push down on your heels. Hold. With each out breath sink lower into your heels and concentrate on lengthening the spine. Slowly return to the starting position. Repeat stretch five times.

BENEFITS...Vitality and youthfulness quickly return when the spine is lengthened in this manner. Adds the spring back into the spine.

TO BEGIN...Lie on your back, bend both knees toward the chest and clasp both knees with both hands...and relax.

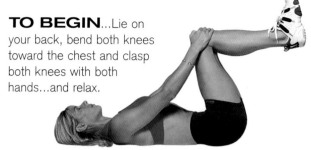

THE STRETCH...Inhale...Exhale...Gently pull in both knees towards the chest and at the same time raise the head as though to kiss the knees. Breathe out as you move, not forgetting to tighten your tummy muscles as you exhale. Hold for a moment, return to the starting position. And repeat five times.

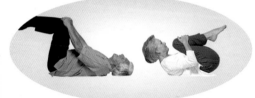

BENEFITS...Feel the stretch in the lower back and buttocks. Regain the feeling of a supple and agile spine. Stretching in this way removes stiffness and restores function.

If it is too hard at first to lift your head, just curl from the lower lumbar, leaving the head resting on the floor.

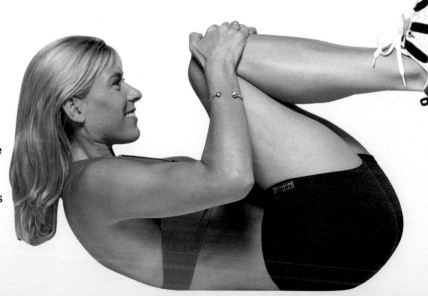

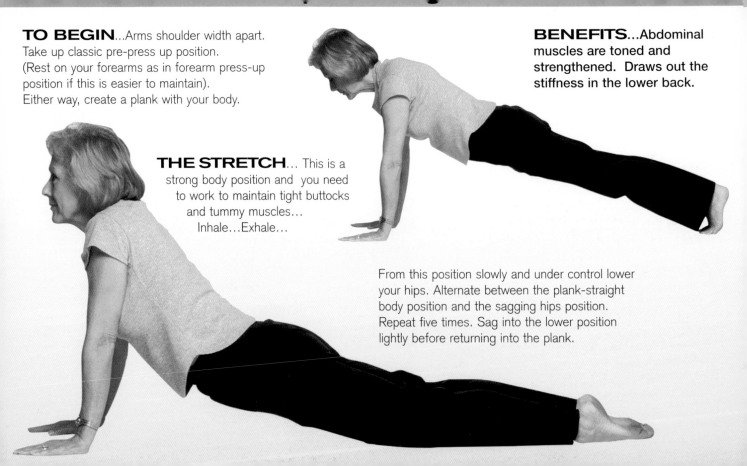

TO BEGIN...Arms shoulder width apart.
Take up classic pre-press up position.
(Rest on your forearms as in forearm press-up
position if this is easier to maintain).
Either way, create a plank with your body.

BENEFITS...Abdominal
muscles are toned and
strengthened. Draws out the
stiffness in the lower back.

THE STRETCH... This is a
strong body position and you need
to work to maintain tight buttocks
and tummy muscles...
Inhale...Exhale...

From this position slowly and under control lower
your hips. Alternate between the plank-straight
body position and the sagging hips position.
Repeat five times. Sag into the lower position
lightly before returning into the plank.

TO BEGIN...Lie flat on the floor on your back, legs straight and arms outstretched above the head.

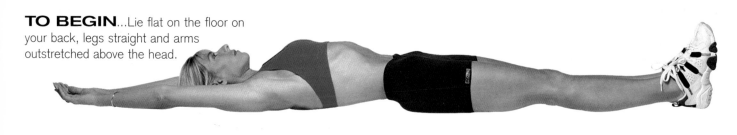

BENEFITS...This stretch is designed to counter poor posture, muscle spasm and restricted movement, allowing the spine once again to function properly. This builds up strength in the neck, which is sadly lacking for most of us.

Sharron's flexibility is amazing, as you can imagine. Do not get discouraged if your movement is more restricted when starting. Practice makes perfect.

THE STRETCH...Inhale...Exhale... Keeping the heels, bottom and head on the floor, raise the chest allowing the shoulders to come away from the floor. Hold for a moment. Lower and relax. Repeat the movement five times.

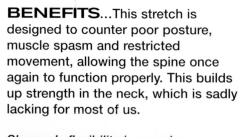

TO BEGIN...Lie face down. Arms out stretched to the side. Palms facing down, body flat, legs together. Lightly resting forehead on the floor.

These stretches are designed to be performed fully clothed and in the comfort of your home.

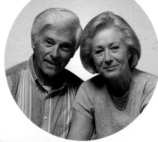

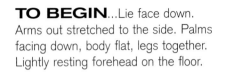

THE STRETCH...Inhale...Exhale...Lift both hands and arms off the ground. Hold. And slowly lower to the starting position. Concentrate on drawing the hands high and away from the body. Repeat five times.

BENEFITS...Squeezes the upper back and shoulder muscles into life.

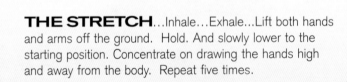

TO BEGIN...Lie flat on your back, knees bent and feet flat on the floor. Wrap your arms around you so your fingertips are touching your shoulder blades. The elbows should be pointing up to the ceiling. Hold and squeeze for a moment.

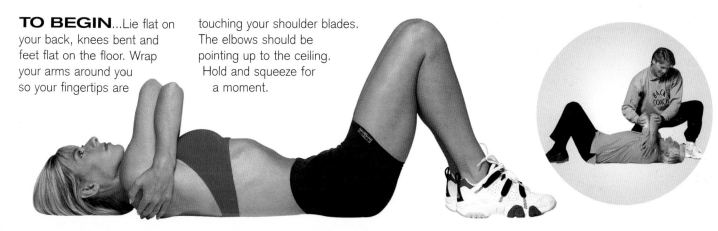

THE STRETCH...Inhale...Exhale...Tighten your tummy muscles, now keeping your feet still and your legs and pelvis stationary, rock/sway your elbows from side to side. Keep looking up to the ceiling.

BENEFITS...You should feel a gentle massaging effect across the upper back and shoulders. This stretch promotes a healthy relaxed back, posturally aligned and moving as nature intended. Just squeezing creates a fantastic release in deep-seated muscle tension.

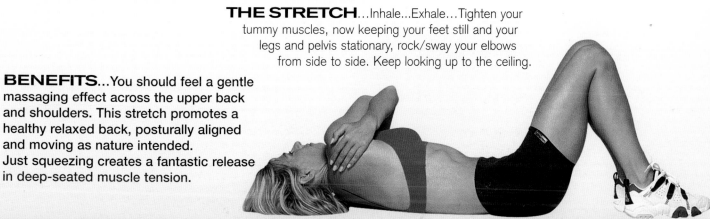

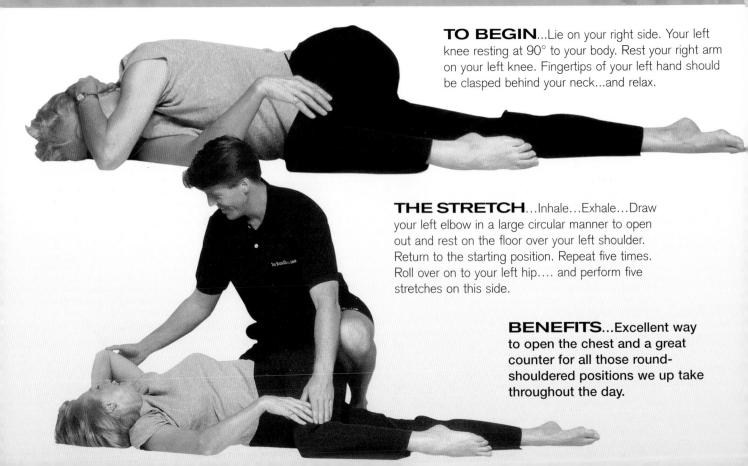

TO BEGIN...Lie on your right side. Your left knee resting at 90° to your body. Rest your right arm on your left knee. Fingertips of your left hand should be clasped behind your neck...and relax.

THE STRETCH...Inhale...Exhale...Draw your left elbow in a large circular manner to open out and rest on the floor over your left shoulder. Return to the starting position. Repeat five times. Roll over on to your left hip.... and perform five stretches on this side.

BENEFITS...Excellent way to open the chest and a great counter for all those round-shouldered positions we up take throughout the day.

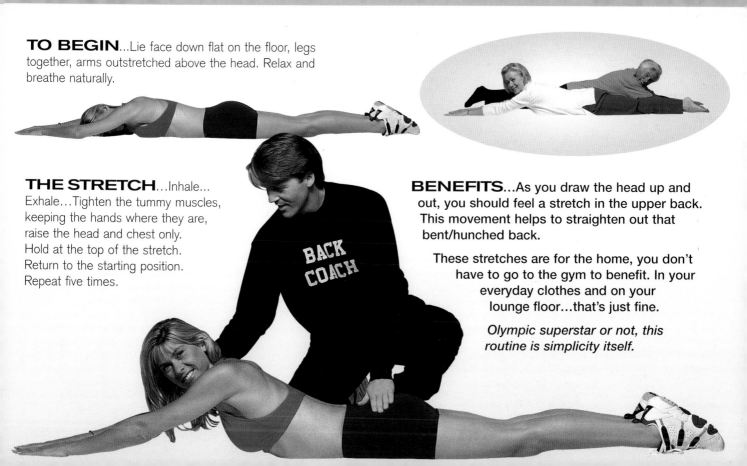

TO BEGIN...Lie face down flat on the floor, legs together, arms outstretched above the head. Relax and breathe naturally.

THE STRETCH...Inhale... Exhale...Tighten the tummy muscles, keeping the hands where they are, raise the head and chest only. Hold at the top of the stretch. Return to the starting position. Repeat five times.

BACK COACH

BENEFITS...As you draw the head up and out, you should feel a stretch in the upper back. This movement helps to straighten out that bent/hunched back.

These stretches are for the home, you don't have to go to the gym to benefit. In your everyday clothes and on your lounge floor...that's just fine.

Olympic superstar or not, this routine is simplicity itself.

TO BEGIN…Lie on your back, knees bent, feet flat on the floor and slightly apart, arms outstretched above your head. Look straight up at the ceiling.

BENEFITS…You will feel a slight release in muscle tension as the floor applies pressure to those tight shoulder muscles. Tuck the chin in to allow the neck to flatten. Feel the arms stretching away from the pelvis. The beauty of these exercises is that they can be easily performed by anyone from superstar athletes to grandparents.

THE STRETCH…Breathe in, and then out as you slowly raise your pelvis to lift the hips off the floor tightening your buttocks and tummy as you do so. Keep your weight on the heels and shoulders to form a bridge. Hold for a moment, breathing naturally, and relax, then return to the starting position. Repeat five times.

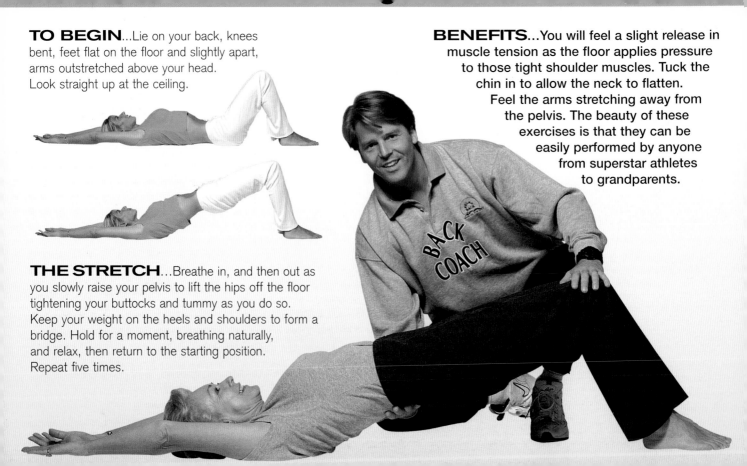

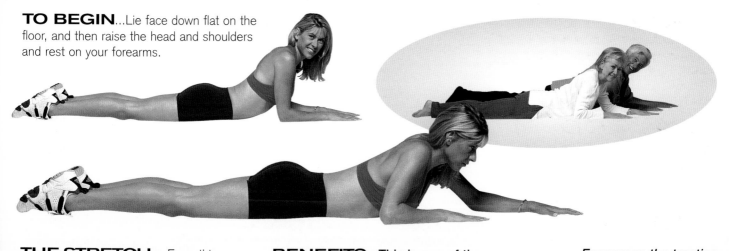

TO BEGIN...Lie face down flat on the floor, and then raise the head and shoulders and rest on your forearms.

THE STRETCH ...From this position inch forward one forearm after the other, drawing yourself forward as if crawling on your forearms. Relax the legs. The hips rotate from side to side.

BENEFITS...This is one of the best ways to stretch the spine. Stretching lengthways eases the joints away from each other, keeping things open and functioning as they were designed.

Encourage the traction effect by allowing the legs to drag 'dead weight' behind as you crawl forward.

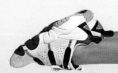

TO BEGIN...Lie flat on your back, legs apart and straight, the arms out to the side at shoulder level, palms upwards.

THE STRETCH...Leaving your right arm flat on the floor, bring your left hand across your chest and slide it down your right arm, twisting at the shoulders. Looking towards your hands, place the palms together. Try to keep your bottom in contact with the floor. Hold this position for a moment, and then return to your starting position. Breathe naturally throughout. Repeat this movement to the other side. Perform five times on both sides.

BENEFITS...This spinal twist releases muscle tension in the upper back and shoulder region, helping you to re-align your posture.

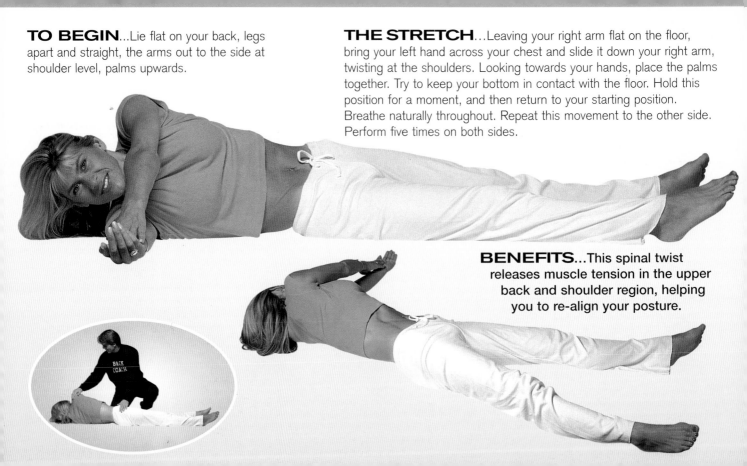

TO BEGIN...Kneeling, sit on your heels. Curl forward to place your forehead as close to the floor near your knees as you can, arms outstretched in front, and palms flat on the floor.

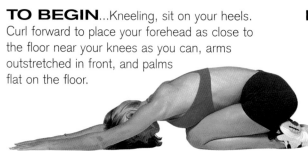

BENEFITS...This stretch opens up and de-squashes the spine. As you relax further into this stretch, feel the spine lengthen from the pelvis to the head. The tightness in the lower back is released.

Each time you breathe out feel yourself sink further into deep relaxation.

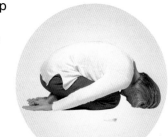

THE STRETCH...As you become more relaxed, take a deep breath in, breathe out and sweep the arms around until the backs of the hands are on the floor near your heels. And relax. Remain in this position for several minutes.

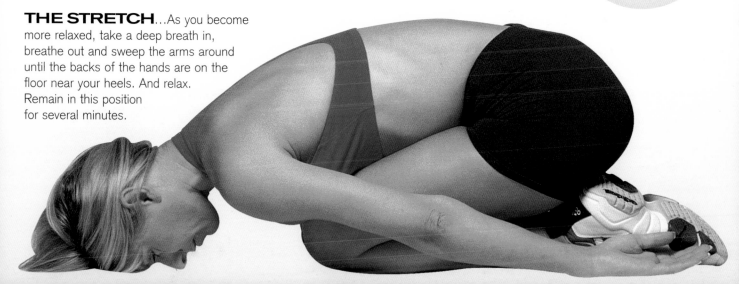

TO BEGIN...Lie on your back, your right arm outstretched over your head. Left arm is relaxed by your side. Stretch out your left leg and bend your right knee, keeping the sole of your right foot flat on the floor.

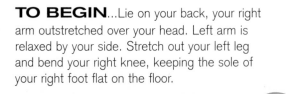

THE STRETCH...Breathe in...Exhale...And now try to stretch the right arm and the left leg further away from the body. Remember to tighten your tummy muscles. Stretch out, hold for a count of three and relax. Do this movement five times. Do the same stretch the other way round, with the left arm and right leg extended, and the right arm and left leg relaxed. Hold for a count of three and relax. Do this movement five times.

BENEFITS...This movement creates a subtle rotation, which you will feel around the pelvis. As you stretch away with arm and leg, try to develop the feeling that these limbs are lengthening.

Never force or strain movements. Stretch as far as you comfortably can and relax. Relaxing in this way takes absolutely no effort.

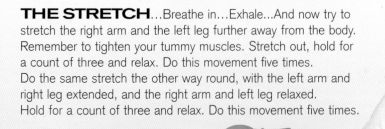

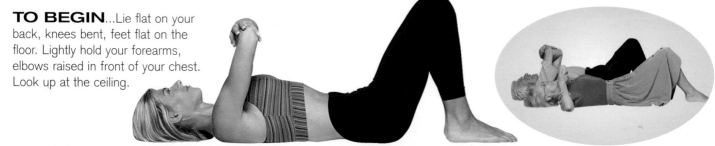

TO BEGIN...Lie flat on your back, knees bent, feet flat on the floor. Lightly hold your forearms, elbows raised in front of your chest. Look up at the ceiling.

THE STRETCH...Inhale...Exhale...Tighten your tummy muscles. Sway the arms over to the right until the right elbow and the back of the right arm are resting gently on the floor. And relax. Inhale... Exhale. Now sway the arms in the other direction. Move smoothly back through the starting position, all the way until the left upper arm and elbow are resting on the floor. And relax. Repeat this sequence five times.

BENEFITS...You should feel the dead weight of the arms subtly stretch the back and shoulders. In this position the weight has been taken off the intervertebral spaces. Relieved of pressure the discs can re-hydrate, repair, and recover. As the back loosens up, it eventually stretches its way to its natural pain-free position.

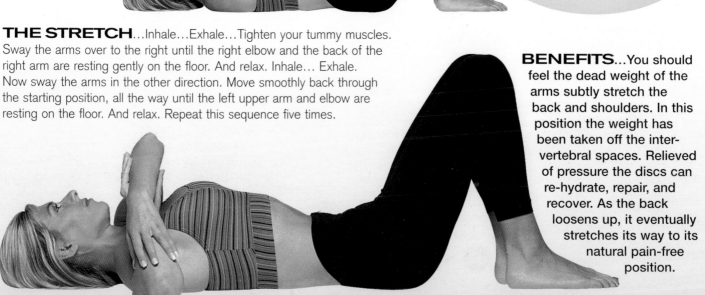

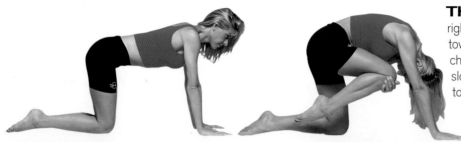

TO BEGIN...Kneel on all fours, with your weight evenly distributed between your hands and knees. Hands should be shoulder width apart, knees slightly apart.

THE STRETCH...Take hold of your right knee with your left hand. Curl your head towards your chest and pull your knee into the chest. Hold for a moment, then uncurl outwards, slowly extending the right leg until it is horizontal to the floor. At the same time extend the left hand horizontally out in front. This movement should be performed slowly and in a controlled manner. Make sure to keep your back in a straight line. The hand, head and foot should be in a straight line and not arched. Return to the starting position and repeat with the other hand and knee. Perform the sequence five times on both sides.

BENEFITS...Try to feel the buttocks relax in the curled position, and tighten them in the uncurled straight body positions. This stretch ensures the discs are maintained in good health by allowing them to move freely.

If you find it too difficult to balance at first, keep both hands on the floor and move the leg only, until you have strengthened your back and have got accustomed to this movement.

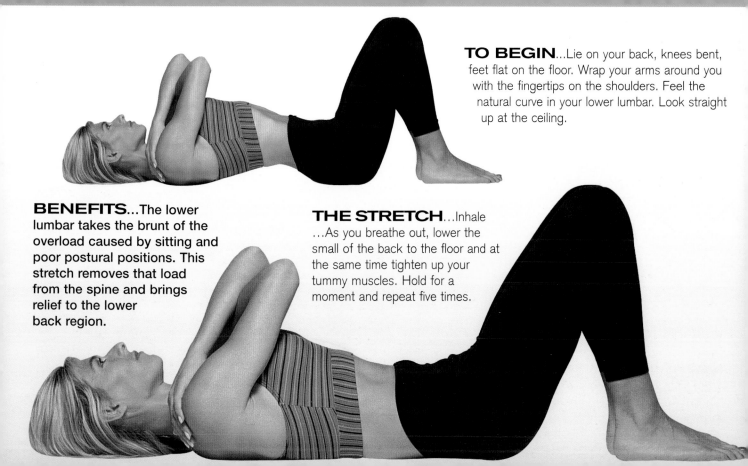

TO BEGIN...Lie on your back, knees bent, feet flat on the floor. Wrap your arms around you with the fingertips on the shoulders. Feel the natural curve in your lower lumbar. Look straight up at the ceiling.

BENEFITS...The lower lumbar takes the brunt of the overload caused by sitting and poor postural positions. This stretch removes that load from the spine and brings relief to the lower back region.

THE STRETCH...Inhale ...As you breathe out, lower the small of the back to the floor and at the same time tighten up your tummy muscles. Hold for a moment and repeat five times.

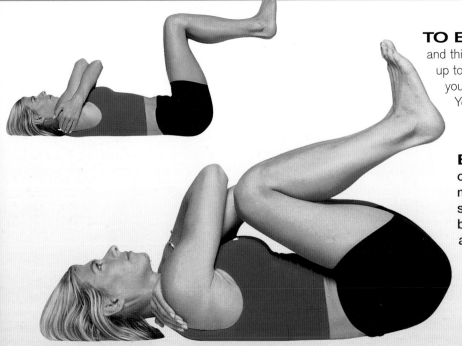

TO BEGIN...Lie flat on your back, knees bent, and thighs perpendicular to the floor and toes pointing up to the ceiling. Wrap your arms around you so your fingertips are touching your shoulder blades. Your elbows should be pointing up to the ceiling.

BENEFITS...This is a subtle stretch of the lower lumbar, and the rocking motion massages the back. Strong stomach muscles are not only important because they make you look good, but also they are essential for keeping a pain-free back.

THE STRETCH...Breathe in, and as you breathe out, rock the legs slightly towards your head, and use your tummy muscles to draw your knees closer to your chest. Lift the pelvis to round the lower lumbar. Repeat five times. Slowly lower the legs...and relax.

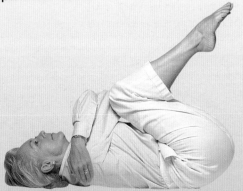

TO BEGIN...Lie flat on your back, knees bent, head resting in a comfortable position and relaxed, arms by your side. Feel the natural curve in your neck.

BENEFITS...
You should feel the neck lengthen. This is a perfect exercise for releasing muscle tension associated with headaches. It helps to loosen up the neck and restores its 'give' and shock absorbing qualities.

This exercise helps strengthen what is essentially a weak body part for the majority of us.

THE STRETCH...Inhale...Exhale... And as you do so, retract the chin and flatten the back of the neck against the floor. Hold for a moment and relax. Repeat five times.

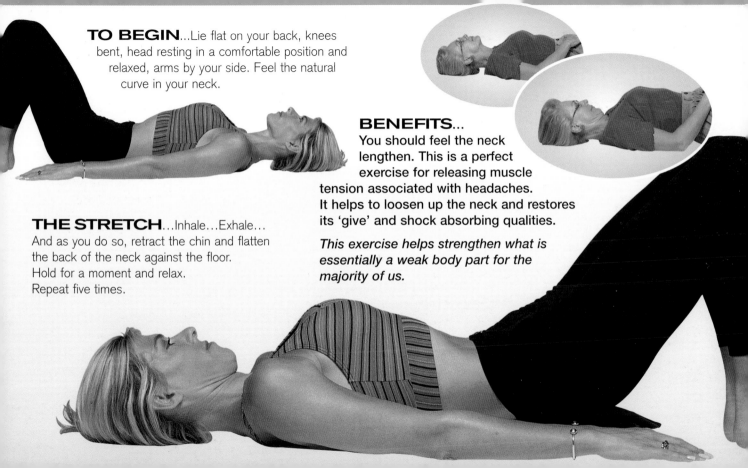

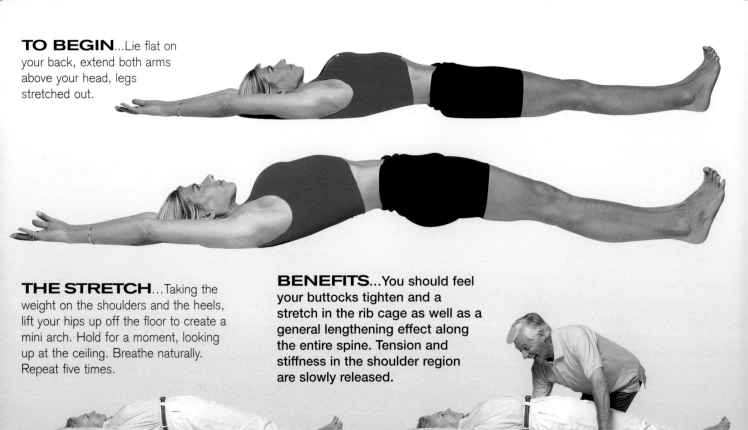

TO BEGIN...Lie flat on your back, extend both arms above your head, legs stretched out.

THE STRETCH...Taking the weight on the shoulders and the heels, lift your hips up off the floor to create a mini arch. Hold for a moment, looking up at the ceiling. Breathe naturally. Repeat five times.

BENEFITS...You should feel your buttocks tighten and a stretch in the rib cage as well as a general lengthening effect along the entire spine. Tension and stiffness in the shoulder region are slowly released.

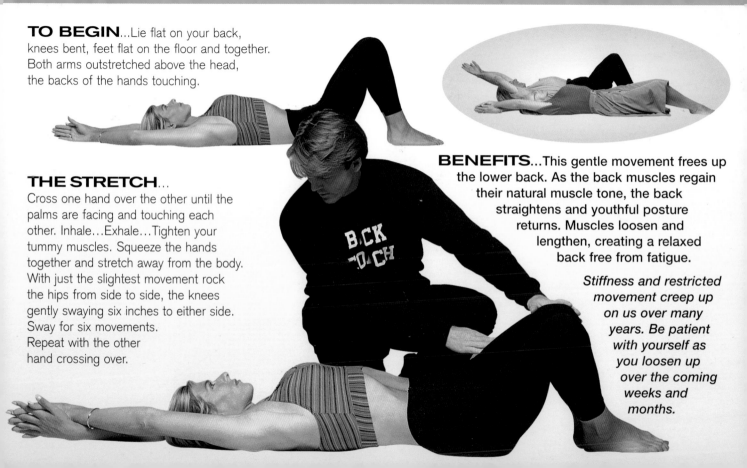

TO BEGIN...Lie flat on your back, knees bent, feet flat on the floor and together. Both arms outstretched above the head, the backs of the hands touching.

THE STRETCH...

Cross one hand over the other until the palms are facing and touching each other. Inhale...Exhale...Tighten your tummy muscles. Squeeze the hands together and stretch away from the body. With just the slightest movement rock the hips from side to side, the knees gently swaying six inches to either side. Sway for six movements. Repeat with the other hand crossing over.

BENEFITS...This gentle movement frees up the lower back. As the back muscles regain their natural muscle tone, the back straightens and youthful posture returns. Muscles loosen and lengthen, creating a relaxed back free from fatigue.

Stiffness and restricted movement creep up on us over many years. Be patient with yourself as you loosen up over the coming weeks and months.

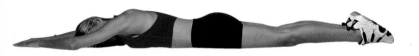

TO BEGIN...Lie face down, lightly resting your forehead on the floor. Legs together, arms outstretched above the head...and relax.

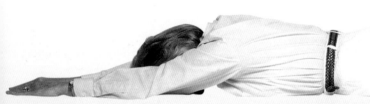

THE STRETCH...Inhale...Exhale...Keeping the head still raise the hands and arms off the floor. Hold at the height of the stretch for 3 seconds. Return arms slowly and under control to starting position. Repeat three times. (As you lift your arms draw the hands away from the body, stretch the fingers away to encourage the lengthening of the spine.)

BENEFITS...This is a great antidote for too much desk work or driving. The effect is to release deep-seated muscle tension in the upper back and shoulders helping to bring back life and energy where fatigue and tension had squeezed it out. Feel the shoulders relax once you return to the floor.

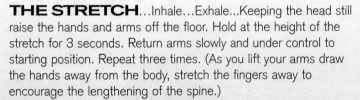

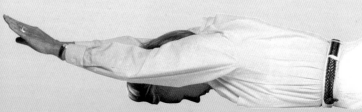

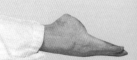

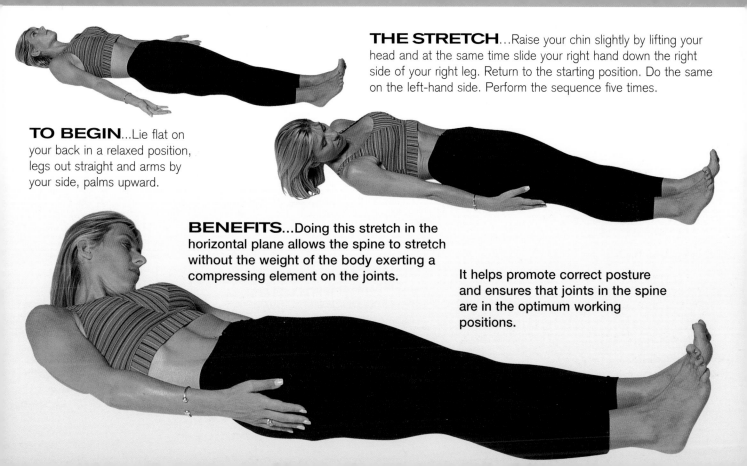

THE STRETCH...Raise your chin slightly by lifting your head and at the same time slide your right hand down the right side of your right leg. Return to the starting position. Do the same on the left-hand side. Perform the sequence five times.

TO BEGIN...Lie flat on your back in a relaxed position, legs out straight and arms by your side, palms upward.

BENEFITS...Doing this stretch in the horizontal plane allows the spine to stretch without the weight of the body exerting a compressing element on the joints.

It helps promote correct posture and ensures that joints in the spine are in the optimum working positions.

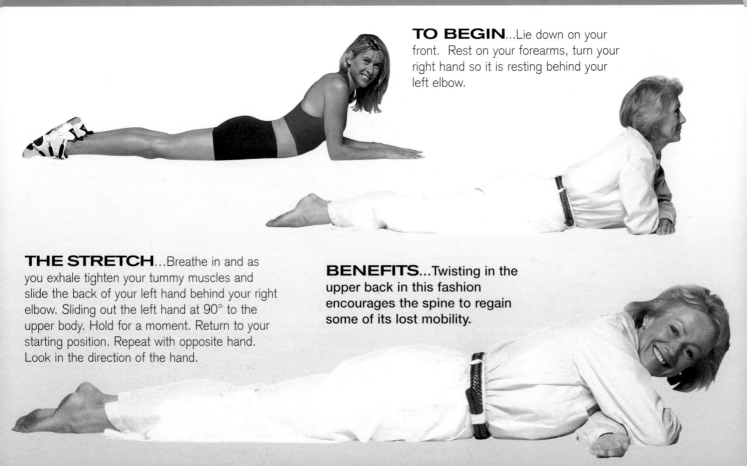

TO BEGIN...Lie down on your front. Rest on your forearms, turn your right hand so it is resting behind your left elbow.

THE STRETCH...Breathe in and as you exhale tighten your tummy muscles and slide the back of your left hand behind your right elbow. Sliding out the left hand at 90° to the upper body. Hold for a moment. Return to your starting position. Repeat with opposite hand. Look in the direction of the hand.

BENEFITS...Twisting in the upper back in this fashion encourages the spine to regain some of its lost mobility.

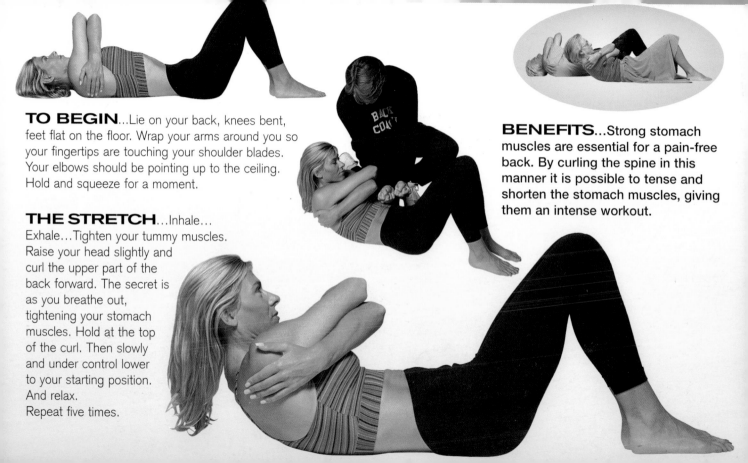

TO BEGIN...Lie on your back, knees bent, feet flat on the floor. Wrap your arms around you so your fingertips are touching your shoulder blades. Your elbows should be pointing up to the ceiling. Hold and squeeze for a moment.

THE STRETCH...Inhale... Exhale...Tighten your tummy muscles. Raise your head slightly and curl the upper part of the back forward. The secret is as you breathe out, tightening your stomach muscles. Hold at the top of the curl. Then slowly and under control lower to your starting position. And relax. Repeat five times.

BENEFITS...Strong stomach muscles are essential for a pain-free back. By curling the spine in this manner it is possible to tense and shorten the stomach muscles, giving them an intense workout.

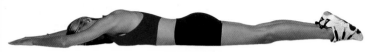

TO BEGIN...Lie face down. Rest your right cheek on the floor. Arms outstretched, draw your arms down until they are out to the side, palms facing downwards.

BENEFITS...Long-term shoulder restrictions have an opportunity to free themselves. Great upper back muscle tension releaser. After a few hours in front of the TV or computer screen this stretch is ideal.

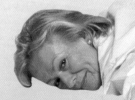

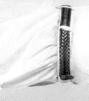

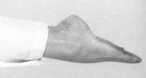

THE STRETCH...Inhale...Exhale...And raise the right hand off the ground. Hold for a moment. And lower the hand back to the ground under control. Inhale...Exhale and raise the hand you are looking at off the ground. (In this case the left hand.) Hold for a moment. And lower. Place your left cheek on the floor.... Inhale.... Exhale and raise your left hand off the floor. Hold for a moment. And lower. Inhale...Exhale and raise the hand you are looking at off the ground. (This time the right hand is raised.) Hold. Lower. Repeat the whole cycle three times.